M000119105

THE LITTLE BOOK OF
RUNNING

Published by OH!
20 Mortimer Street
London W1T 3JW

ISBN 978-1-80069-005-9

Compiled by: Chas Newkey-Burden
Editorial: Lisa Dyer
Project manager: Russell Porter
Design: Andy Jones
Production: Freencky Portas

A CIP catalogue record for this book is available from the British Library

Printed in Dubai

10 9 8 7 6 5 4 3 2 1

Illustrations: Freepik.com

THE LITTLE BOOK OF

RUNNING

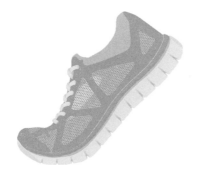

FOR EVERYONE FROM
THE BEGINNER TO
THE LONG-DISTANCE RUNNER

CONTENTS

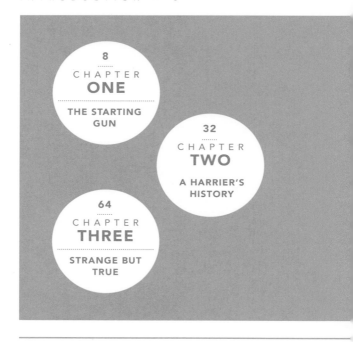

INTRODUCTION

Why do people choose to run? Whether it is for physical fitness, to boost mental health or simply for a bit of "me time", there are many benefits to this increasingly popular form of exercise. If you want to improve as a runner, then understanding more about your favourite pastime will help you stand out from the pack.

You'll learn lots of detailed information in the pages ahead, together with inspirational and amusing quotes about running. Take a trot through the history of the sport, from ancient Greece to the digital age of jogging apps and Parkrun, discover some of the world's strangest marathons and read stories of remarkable endurance.

With plenty to amuse and inspire any runner, this book contains a marathon worth of facts and fun wrapped up in a five-kilometre package. You will discover the relationship between Oscar Wilde and the treadmill, find out why your nipples are bleeding and pick up tips on how to run faster without it hurting.

Running builds bone, strengthens muscle, improves heart health and burns calories. It encourages better sleep and a more positive mental attitude. It is a hobby that brings health and joy to all who take part in it. Keep this book handy and you can get even more of both from your daily run.

CHAPTER
ONE

THE STARTING GUN

Are you ready for the miles ahead? Finish your stretching, get your running shoes on and pace your way through these opening facts and stats. There's quite an interesting road ahead, so let's set out now…

Some 6.8 million people in the UK and 60 million in the USA are regular runners. Improving fitness is the primary motivation for taking up the exercise.

Source: Statista.com

The youngest marathon runner in the world is Budhia Singh – he completed 48 marathons before his fifth birthday.

The running community is highly active on social media and connects runners from around the world.

To date, more than 70 million posts are tagged #running on Instagram.

Source: Instagram.com

Some experts say stretching before a run is best, while others say it is better to stretch after a run. But a few recent studies report that any stretching can do more harm than good.

A good answer is to listen to your body.

Source: National Library of Medicine

Over one billion pairs of
running shoes are sold
worldwide every year – out of
an estimated 19 billion pairs
of shoes overall.

Sources: Sportskeeda.com and WorldFootwear.com

The first international Parkrun – the 5 kilometre (3.1 mile) race – was held at Bushy Park in London, England, in 2004.

The first international event launched in Zimbabwe in 2007. It now takes place every Saturday at 2,000 locations in 22 countries across five continents.

You take an average of 50 breaths a minute when you run, as opposed to 15 when you rest. This is so your body can keep up with the demand for more oxygen and increased carbon dioxide production.

Source: National Institutes of Health

With the London Monopoly Running Challenge, joggers see how many London Monopoly streets and stations they can visit (or "buy") in 60 minutes.

Each location has a monetary value so you can keep track of your accumulating riches.

Source: RunnersGuidetoLondon.co.uk

The first New York City marathon was held in 1970, there were 127 registered runners and the entry fee was just one dollar.

By 2019, there were over 54,000 runners with all 50 states and over 140 countries represented.

Source: New York Road Runners

Funny names for running clubs around the world include *Agony of Defeet, Easier Said than Run* and *We've Got the Runs.*

In 1967 Kathrine Switzer made history as the first woman to run the Boston Marathon, having entered under her initials and surname only as females were prohibited. An official tried unsuccessfully to eject her mid-race. It wasn't until 1972 that the Boston Marathon officially admitted women.

Source: The Association of International Marathons and Distance Races

Some runners notice their performance and enthusiasm rise when they have a running partner with whom to pound the pavements.

Others prefer a virtual running partner – a person they share their distances, speeds and experiences with online.

To help you achieve good posture as you run, many coaches recommend that you imagine you are trying to carry a potato chip in each hand without crushing it.

Source: RunnersWorld.com

Carb-loading is the practice of eating extra portions of carbohydrates to bolster your reserves ahead of a long run. It maximizes glycogen stores, which help delay fatigue and optimize performance.

Source: RunnersWorld.com

Endurance events deliberately held in particularly muddy and hazardous conditions are known as "muddy runs".

A split is the time recorded for any specific segment of a run.

Runners use splits to check that they are pacing evenly and staying on track to meet their goal.

As much as 70 per cent of runners will sustain an injury at some point.

Knee injuries are the most common, but other injuries affecting runners include Achilles tendinitis, shin splints, heel pain and torn muscles.

Source: American Academy of Physical Medicine and Rehabilitation

Not everyone is capable of running a marathon in a good time. In fact, 20 per cent of people won't achieve this no matter how hard they train as their muscles aren't genetically programmed to extract as much oxygen as they need.

Source: Loughborough University

A study for the University of Arkansas found that 80 per cent of men and 60 per cent of women felt more attractive due to regular running.

Source: *Running: Cheaper Than Therapy* (Bloomsbury, 2017)

Researchers who studied 300,000 Chicago marathon participants found that women are more likely to negative split than men because they run more conservatively in the first half.

Source: RuntotheFinish.com

Spanish researchers found
that men run their fastest
marathon at age 27, while
women peak at 29.

Times were four per cent slower
for every year younger than
these ages, and became two
per cent slower for each
year thereafter.

Source: BMC Sports Science, Medicine
and Rehabilitation

The Walt Disney World Marathon is held at Disney theme parks, with a route lined by Disney characters and Mickey Mouse finisher medals handed to all who complete the course.

CHAPTER
TWO

A HARRIER'S HISTORY

From its roots in ancient Greece,
running has evolved at quite a pace.
Well, we suppose it would have! From
the invention of the stopwatch to
historic, record-breaking moments
to the first-ever marathon, the story
of running is quite breathtaking.

The starting point for running as a sport is 776 BCE, in the town of Olympia, ancient Greece.

The first event in the first Olympics was a race called the stadion, named after the building in which it took place.

The 100 metre distance of today's Olympic race is believed to be the modern-day equivalent of the stadion sprint of ancient Greece, which was about 180 metres (200 yards).

The stopwatch was invented
in 1776, by Frenchman
Jean-Moyes Pouzai, who called
it the chronograph.

At the end of the 17th century, British aristocrats began to employ footmen, who ran and walked long distances, to carry letters and bring back replies.

Some employers placed bets on who would prove superior in a race trial.

Running shoes were invented in the 1800s.

In 1832, Wait Webster patented the process of attaching rubber soles to the shoes, paving the way for plimsolls, or sneakers.

In 1852, the first running spikes were added.

On 6 May 1954, Roger Bannister, a student, ran a mile in 3:59.4 at the Iffley Road track at Oxford University.

He became the first human to run a sub-four-minute mile.

In May 1954, Diane Leather from Staffordshire, England, became the first woman to run a mile in under five minutes at 4:59.23, 23 days after Roger Bannister's sub-four-minute mile.

The winner of the first modern-day marathon in 1896 was a Greek water-carrier named Spyridon Louis, who completed the distance in 2 hours 58 minutes and 50 seconds.

The Boston Marathon was launched in April 1897, in response to the enthusiasm generated by the 1896 Summer Olympics in Athens, Greece.

In the USA, jogging was originally known as "roadwork", so-called because it was part of an athlete's training programme to run several miles every day.

Arthur Leslie Lydiard, the New Zealand runner and athletics coach, is widely credited with popularizing the sport of running across the world, largely due to his promotion of running for health as well as his endurance base-training methods.

What has become known as the East African Running Revolution began in 1968 when Kip Keino, a Kenyan, defeated Jim Ryun (the world record holder) for Gold in the 1500 metre race at the Olympic Games.

In 1966, a book called *Jogging* was published in the US, which helped make the pastime popular.

During the 1970s, it is estimated that 25 million Americans took up running, including the actor Clint Eastwood and US President Jimmy Carter.

In 1984, Adidas launched a running shoe that included a computer – the Micropacer. It calculated distance, average pace and calories burned.

Usain Bolt, born in Jamaica on 21 August 1986, became the world record holder in the 100 metres, 200 metres and 4 × 100 metres relay. He is widely considered the greatest sprinter of all time.

In 2020, the London Marathon was an elite-only event, due to restrictions caused by the COVID-19 global pandemic, as was the Tokyo Marathon.

Many other marathons around the world were cancelled, postponed or held virtually.

In 2019 there were 715 marathons scheduled around the US – an average of 1.9 per day.

Source: Rockay.com

In the late 19th century, a competitive type of foot-walking, known as "pedestrianism", was very popular as a spectator sport and highly competitive.

The races often covered long distances – what would now be considered ultramarathons.

It is believed that the first official ultramarathon was held in 1926 in Mexico City, Mexico, as part of the Central American Games.

Jogging was so uncommon in the 1960s in the USA that people were stopped by police as they pounded the pavements. These included South Carolina Senator Strom Thurmond, and Dick Cordier, a Connecticut, resident who was given a fine for the "illegal use of a highway by a pedestrian".

Source: Vox.com

The steeplechase, a 3,000 metre course over obstacles such as water ditches and hurdles, dates back to an 1850 cross-country foot race at the University of Oxford.

Source: Britannica.com

In 1981, the first London Marathon was held.

More than 20,000 applied to take part; 6,747 were accepted and 6,255 crossed the finish line.

At the 2012 London Olympic Games, 19-year-old Sarah Attar became the first woman from Saudi Arabia to compete in an Olympic track and field event, running the 800 metres race.

On 2 October 2003, Rosie
Swale-Pope, the first woman to
"run around the world", began
her five-year journey, starting
from her home town of Tenby
in Wales on her 57th birthday,
reaching her finish in New York
City on 2 October 2007.

Parkrun was founded by Paul Sinton-Hewitt on 2 October 2004 at Bushy Park in London.

More than six million runners have since officially taken part in a Parkrun.

In 2005, the average finish time for completing a Parkrun was 22:17. By 2018, it was 32:29, as a wider range of people joined the event.

In 2019, $14,717 million
was spent on running shoes
in the US alone.

Source: Statista.com

The Couch to 5K running plan, which gradually builds up new runners to achieve a five kilometre distance, was created by Josh Clark in 1996. Downloads of the app soared by nearly a million in the UK in 2020 as the nation attempted to shed weight gained in the COVID-19 lockdowns.

Source: Telegraph.co.uk

In 2015, Ben Smith, a 36-year-old man from Portishead in England, sold all his belongings, bought a camper van and set off to run 401 marathons in 401 days, raising £330,000 ($450,000) for charities.

Source: The401Challenge.co.uk

The popularity of extreme running is soaring.

The number of ultramarathons increased 1,000 per cent between 2008 and 2018.

Source: *The Guardian*

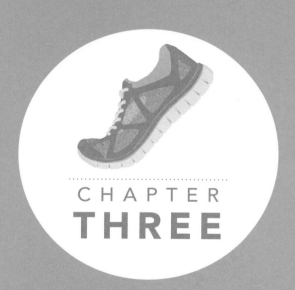

CHAPTER
THREE

STRANGE
BUT TRUE

Did you know running can shave
an inch off your height and get you
high the same way cannabis can?
Or that people have run marathons
in very strange locations, including
outer space? Here are the highs
and lows of the weirder side of
this pastime.

A study published in the *Journal of Cardiovascular Medicine* found that three shots of whisky made no significant difference in treadmill runs.

Source: Telegraph.co.uk

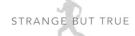

At the World Championship
Pack Burro Race in Fairplay,
Colorado, each runner tackles
the course accompanied by
a donkey bearing a minimum
of 15 kilograms (33 pounds) of
mining gear.

Source: UltraSignup.com

Amusing costumes have become a familiar feature of running events.

Recent events saw people dress up as pink flamingos, bottles of ale, Star Wars stormtroopers and landmarks such as the Eiffel Tower and Big Ben.

Despite poor relations between the two countries, 25 per cent of the foreign runners at the 2014 Pyongyang Marathon in North Korea were Americans.

The Man Versus Horse Marathon takes place in Britain's smallest town, Llanwrtyd Wells in Wales.

A horse won for the first 24 years of the contest, until an elite British marathon runner, Huw Lob, became the race's first human victor.

In September 2020, Brigham Young University runner Whittni Orton broke the world record for running a mile while dribbling a basketball. She completed the curious task in 4:58.56, beating the previous record by ten seconds.

Taking place 200 metres below sea level in the Jordan Valley, along the Sea of Galilee in Israel, the Tiberias Marathon is believed to be the lowest marathon course in the world.

The British explorer and adventurer Sir Ranulph Fiennes ran marathons on seven consecutive days in seven continents in 2003, after a heart attack and bypass operation.

In April 2016, the British astronaut Tim Peake ran the London Marathon on a treadmill in space. He completed the distance in 3:35:21.

In 1983, a 61-year-old Australian farmer called Cliff Young won a 875 kilometre (544 mile) endurance race from Sydney to Melbourne because he ran throughout the night while the younger "professional" athletes slept.

In 2007, three ultra-endurance athletes ran the equivalent of two marathons a day for 111 days to become the first modern runners to cross 7,000 kilometres (4,300 miles) of the Sahara Desert.

Source: RunnersWorld.com

Despite being diagnosed with asthma as a teenager, British long-distance runner Paula Radcliffe went on to win multiple races and championships, and she held the women's world marathon record with a time of 2:15:25 for 16 years.

Source: PaulaRadcliffe.com

The astronaut Sunita Williams took running to another level – she ran the 2007 Boston Marathon onboard the International Space Station, at the same time as her sister and a fellow astronaut were running in it on Earth.

Source: NASA.gov

Haitian runner Dieudonné LaMothe was ordered by his nation's dictator to finish his race or he would be killed. That's motivation for you!

Japanese athlete Shizo Kanakuri was favourite to win the marathon at the 1912 Olympics in Stockholm. He mysteriously disappeared during the race and was listed as a missing person by the Swedish police for the next 50 years…

...It eventually emerged that a heat-exhausted Kanakuri had collapsed and was cared for by a local family. He quietly sailed back to Japan, too embarrassed to admit he had abandoned the race!

In 1967, Kanakuri returned to Sweden and completed the marathon – 54 years after he started it.

A Russian jeweller called Boris Fyodorov completed his first marathon as a solo runner in -38°C (-32.8°F) in 2014.

He took just over five hours to complete the 26.2 miles in the town of Oymyakon.

Source: NBCSports.com

In 2011, Belgian runner Stefaan Engels set the first record for the most consecutive marathons run in a single year – at 365. He was 49 years of age.

A study at the University of Oxford concluded that the post-run buzz people get after running is sparked by cannabinoid receptors – also involved in the marijuana high – in addition to exercise-induced endorphins.

Source: PNAS.org

In 2002, 90-year-old Jenny Wood-Allen became the oldest woman to complete a marathon, finishing the course in 11:34:00.

She took part despite injuring her head in a fall during training.

In Victorian times, alcohol was regarded as a performance enhancer and athletes would drink wine to boost their energy.

Achim Aretz set the world record for the fastest half marathon, running backwards, in 2009 in Essen, Germany. He managed the 21.1 kilometres (13.1 miles) in 1:40:29.

His fellow German, Markus Jürgens, holds the marathon world record in backward running. At the 2017 Hannover Marathon, he crossed the finish line in 3:38:27.

With a whopping 250,000 sweat glands, your feet can produce up to a pint of sweat each day.

Make sure you alternate your running shoes!

Source: Foot.com

Running a marathon can shave up to half an inch off your height because the discs in your back leak water and become shorter under the repetitive strain.

But don't worry – it's only temporary!

A recent survey found that
11 per cent of female Canadian
runners run without underwear,
while just eight per cent of
American women admit
to jogging commando.

Source: RunnersWorld.com

Researchers have found that most runners will straighten up when an attractive runner is approaching them.

Do you find running on a treadmill hard work?

There is a good reason for that: it was originally designed for English prisons as a tool for punishment. Among the inmates to endure this particular form of punishment was Oscar Wilde.

Source: *Smithsonian* magazine

The Tromsø Midnight Sun Marathon takes place in Norway in an evening in June, but because the sun does not set between May and July, the race is held in broad daylight.

Across a range of sports, researchers found that athletes who wear red are more likely to win.

Source: *The New York Times*

In 1986, Vietnam War veteran
Bob Weiland crossed the finish
line of the marathon in four
days, two hours, 47 minutes
and 17 seconds. He had tackled
the entire route on his hands,
having lost his legs in battle
17 years earlier.

In 2017, Harriette Thompson became the oldest woman to finish a half marathon. She was 94 years of age.

If you ran 19.3 kilometres
(12 miles) a day for 2,075 days,
you would complete 40,047
kilometres (24,900 miles) – the
circumference of the planet.

During the Marathon du Médoc, runners have the chance to sample a selection of vinos at the 23 wine tastings along the route. There are also refuelling stations offering oyster, foie gras, cheese and ice cream.

In the US, 43 per cent of runners would rather run on a treadmill than skip a run when the weather is poor.

In Germany, 52 per cent would brave bad weather no matter what.

Source: RunnersWorld.com

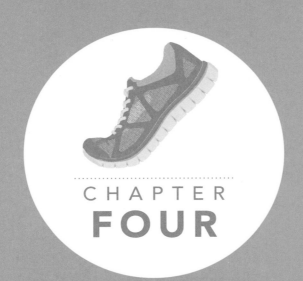

CHAPTER
FOUR

THEY
SAID IT

The wit and wisdom of runners is an
arena all of its own. Whether you
are after motivational soundbites
or gallows humour, you have come
to the right place. On protesting
muscles, punctured egos and inner
peace – here are the words
of the wise.

Lacing up and leaving the house is the hardest moment of any run. You never regret it once you are en route.

Alexandra Heminsley, *Running Like a Girl* (Hutchinson, 2013)

My doctor told me that jogging could add years to my life. I think he was right. I feel ten years older already.

Milton Berle,
as seen on Telegraph.co.uk

Keep listening to your body. It'll tell you when something's not okay.

Emily Infeld,
as seen on RunnersWorld.com

If you are losing faith in human nature, go out and watch a marathon.

Kathrine Switzer,
as seen on WomensHealthMag.com

Years ago, women sat in kitchens
drinking coffee and discussing life.
Today they cover the same topics
while they run.

Joan Benoit Samuelson,
as seen on RunnersWorld.com

THEY SAID IT

66

Run like a millennial runs from
commitment!

99

Spectator sign seen at a marathon

Running is fun. Indulge this instinct. Enjoy it. After all, there aren't many animal impulses that we can act on in public without getting arrested.

Mark Remy,
The Runner's Rule Book (Rodale, 2009)

"

If running taught me anything, it was how to turn things around. So many times I had dreaded a workout, only for it to turn out splendid. So many days I had been convinced I would get lost. Only to be thrilled by new scenery as I found my way.

"

Nita Sweeney,
Depression Hates a Moving Target: How Running with My Dog Brought Me Back from the Brink, (Mango, 2019)

Running is my meditation, mind flush,
cosmic telephone, mood elevator
and spiritual communion.

Lorraine Moller,
as seen on RunnersWorld.com

66

There is nothing quite so gentle,
deep and irrational as running – and
nothing quite so savage, so wild.

99

Bernd Heinrich,
Why We Run: A Natural History
(Harper Collins, 2007)

Running was the thing I could do on my own, with no one to compete against. It cleared my head and stopped me from going bonkers when I was getting up at 4am to present a breakfast show, with all the myopic egotism that can create.

Broadcaster **Sian Williams**,
in *Running: Cheaper Than Therapy*
(Bloomsbury, 2017)

All runners are tough. Everyone has to have a little fire in them, that even in tough times can't be turned off.

Shalane Flanagan,
Olympic long-distance runner,
as seen on WomensHealthMag.com.

If you have a body, you are an athlete.

Bill Bowerman,
co-founder of Nike, as seen on Nike.com

Winning is great, sure, but if you are really going to do something in life, the secret is learning how to lose. Nobody goes undefeated all the time. If you can pick up after a crushing defeat, and go on to win again, you are going to be a champion someday.

Wilma Rudolph,
Olympic sprinter, as seen on
WomensHealthMag.com

Just because your muscles start to protest doesn't mean you have to listen.

Author unknown,
as seen on *Runner's High* calendar

Running is about finding your inner
peace, and so is life well lived.

Dean Karnazes,
as seen on RunnersWorld.com

I always loved running… it was something you could do by yourself and under your own power. You could go in any direction, fast or slow as you wanted, fighting the wind if you felt like it, seeking out new sights just on the strength of your feet and the courage of your lungs.

Jesse Owens,
as seen on TheActiveTimes.com

> Somebody may beat me, but they are going to have to bleed to do it.

Steve Prefontaine,
as seen on RunnersBlueprint.com

I believe that every human has a finite number of heartbeats. I don't intend to waste any of mine running around doing exercises.

Neil Armstrong

As every runner knows, running is about more than just putting one foot in front of the other; it is about our lifestyle and who we are.

Joan Benoit Samuelson,
as seen on RunnersTribe.com

You imagine running 120 miles a week, week in, week out, for the past four or five years. It takes a little bit out of you.

Mo Farah,
as seen in *Men's Health* magazine

"

Jogging is very beneficial. It's good for your legs and your feet. It's also very good for the ground. It makes it feel needed.

"

Charles M. Schultz,
as seen on RuntotheFinish.com

Always give 100 per cent – apart from when giving blood.

Sign seen at a marathon,
as featured in *Running: Cheaper Than Therapy*
(Bloomsbury, 2017)

I'll be happy if running and I can grow old together.

Haruki Murakami,
as seen on ChargeRunning.com

Running is the greatest metaphor
for life, because you get out of
it what you put into it.

Oprah Winfrey,
as seen on Huffingtonpost.co.uk

"

Sure, it's hard and long, but since when has that been a bad thing?

A spectator sign, as seen at the 2017 Dublin Marathon

Running in the middle of the night, it's not ideal.

Colin Johnstone,
who ran marathons starting at 2am during the
COVID-19 lockdown, as seen on BBC.co.uk

I can still push myself in the same way as I get older. I still approach racing and training in the same way. I just have different fitness and time goals in mind.

Deena Kastor,
as seen on RunnersWorld.com

If you want to become the best
runner you can be, start now.
Don't spend the rest of your life
wondering if you can do it.

Priscilla Welch,
in *The Quotable Runner* (Breakaway Books, 2001)

Don't dream of winning,
train for it.

Mo Farah,
as seen on AZQuotes.com

Dancing and running shake the chemistry of happiness.

Matthew Coley, aphorist, as seen on Amazon.co.uk

We are designed to run and we increase our chances of happiness when we do so.

Jeff Galloway, running coach, as seen on JeffGalloway.com

A lot of people run a race to see who's the fastest. I run to see who has the most guts.

Steve Prefontaine,
as seen on RunnerBlueprint.com

66

Every major decision I've made in
the last eight years has been prefaced
by a run.

99

Casey Neistat, filmmaker,
as seen on RunnersWorld.com

CHAPTER
FIVE

HINTS
AND TIPS

If you are interested in improving
your finish time or simply want to
enjoy and understand running better,
feast your eyes on these fascinating
facts, tips and hints.

To avoid cramping and digestive troubles, wait for about two hours after a main meal before your run.

Don't eat or drink anything new,
or wear a new kit, on race day.

Studies have shown that running for up to 60 minutes at a moderate intensity can bolster your immune system by accelerating the circulation of protective antibodies.

Interval runs – consisting of
a mixture of fast and slow
segments – are named *fartleks*,
after a Swedish word meaning
"speed play".

In a study for the University of California, people who began to run four times a week reported a 30 per cent increase in the amount of sex they had.

Source: RunnersWorld.com

A study for the journal *Medicine and Science in Sports and Exercise* found that sleeping an extra 75 minutes on six consecutive nights ahead of a marathon can help your performance on the day.

Source: ACSM.org

The prolonged chaffing that running can cause sometimes leads to bleeding nipples, a condition known as "jogger's nipple". Applying an adhesive bandage or anti-chafing balm can help.

Ever been caught short during a run?

You're not alone: the jostling motion can cause muscle contractions in the intestines, moving whatever you have eaten along the tract.

Your feet swell as you run, which can lead to your toes rubbing against the top of your shoes.

This can eventually create blood blisters beneath the toenails, giving the appearance of black nails.

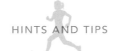

Listening to music can boost your running performance by up to 15 per cent.

Source: RunSociety.com

In 2016, the *Journal of the American Medical Association* stated that high-fitness exercisers, including runners, had a lower risk for developing 26 different kinds of cancer than those who do little or no exercise.

Source: JAMANetwork.com

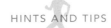
Aerobic exercise such as running can improve cognitive function and reduce the incidence of cognitive decline and Alzheimer's, according to *Current Alzheimer Research.*

Source: BenthamScience.com

You should eat within two hours of finishing a run, because this is when your muscles are best able to replenish their glycogen stores.

According to a recent survey, people who post their runs on social media are more likely to run 5 kilometres (3 miles) in a quicker time than those who do not.

Source: RunnersRadar.com

When you run, you use 26 bones, 33 joints, 112 ligaments and countless nerves, tendons and blood vessels.

Source: AAPSM.org

On average, professional runners take 185 to 200 steps per minute.

The risk of running-related injuries increases significantly after 45 years of age.

The remedy?

Strength training will help you stay strong and prevent muscle mass from declining.

Source: RunnersWorld.com

Once runners hit their 70s, they are likely to notice a decline in performance.

Source: *Masters Athletes: A Model for Healthy Aging*, University of Pittsburgh

Want to lose weight?

By running in the morning, you will get your metabolism fired up and burn more calories during the rest of the day.

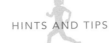

A one-hour run adds seven hours to your life, according to the journal *Progress in Cardiovascular Diseases*.

Source: Journals.Elsevier.com

Do you find you cough after
finishing a run?

You are probably suffering from
bronchoconstriction: a spasm
that attacks the small muscles
lining your lungs.

Another common symptom after running is "brain fog".

This happens because the exertion, especially in very prolonged exercise, has depleted your glycogen, leaving your brain short of fuel.

Source: National Institutes of Health

The American College of Cardiology estimates that the chance of suffering a heart attack during a marathon is one in 75,1000.

A study from Boston University found that regular running improves knee health and strengthens bones and joints.

Dress for how warm you will feel one mile into the run – not how warm you will feel as you first leave the house.

The most effective training sessions mimic the event for which you're training.

Want to run a 5K at a sub-eight-minute pace? Make sure you run at that pace on your training runs.

Want to avoid injury?

Make sure you never increase weekly training mileage by more than 10 per cent per week.

Build up to and complete at
least one 32 kilometre (20 mile)
training run before a marathon.

If you want the endorphins that make you feel high after a run, then make sure you push yourself a bit… but not too much! Otherwise you might just feel drained.

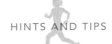

Doing other forms of training as well as running will help you avoid injury.

Cycling, swimming or strength-training are popular.

Studies show that running uphill slows you down more than running downhill speeds you up.

For each mile that you run at a race or official event, allow one day of recovery before returning to hard training or racing.

Running regularly is great.

Running every day is counter-
productive and could be
dangerous, as you're not giving
your body the time and fuel it
needs to go through adaptation
– the building of mitochondria,
blood vessels and muscle fibres.

If you're just getting started in running, don't set out to reach your goal in one non-stop run. Break the run down into intervals, and walk for a minute or two between the intervals.

Keep training this way until you can run the entire distance without stopping.

CHAPTER
SIX

THE
FINISHING LINE

The end is in sight and your sweaty
body will be relieved to complete
this journey. Before you cross the
finishing line, here is a final kilometre
of facts for you. From running movies
to anaerobic thresholds and final-mile
heroics, this chapter will see you reach
your goal.

The marathon was first designated its course for the 1908 Olympic Games.

The British royal family requested that it start at Windsor Castle and end at the Olympic Stadium's royal box – a distance of 26.2 miles.

Humans create fewer new brain cells as we age but a study at Cambridge University found that regular running can reverse this development.

Source: Telegraph.co.uk

Running stimulates brain cell growth, particularly in the hippocampus region, which is linked to memory and learning.

The oldest person to run a mile under four minutes was Eamonn Coghlan of Ireland, who was 41 when he ran 3:58.15.

A study found that those who run in the open air show higher post-workout self-esteem than those who work out in the gym.

Source: *Psychology Today*

A study at Rhode Island College found that running boosts creativity and concentration.

A study in the *American Journal of Cardiology* found a strong link between running endurance, and sexual endurance.

Source: RunnersBlueprint.com

Several films have been made about running, including *Chariots of Fire* (1981), *The Loneliness of the Long Distance Runner* (1962) and *Run Fatboy Run* (2007).

Running can help you live longer.

Researchers tracked 138 healthy, first-time marathon runners and found that training for and completing the London marathon caused a four-year reduction in their overall "vascular age".

Source: BBC.co.uk

Women burn around 75 per cent more fat than men while running.

Source: *The Complete Book of Running for Women* (Gallery Books, 2000)

Most runners complete a marathon in between four and five hours, with an average mile time of 9 to 11.5 minutes.

Running helps those suffering from post-traumatic stress disorder (PTSD), according to a study in the *Journal of Psychiatric Research.*

Source: Journals.Elsevier.com

Running in the afternoon when your body temperature is higher will help you perform better.

A major gripe among participants at marathons and other racing events is when a runner suddenly stops in celebration at the finishing line, causing a pile-up of runners.

Your anaerobic threshold is the stage in your run when lactic acid buildup causes exhaustion. It is also sometimes known as the "lactate threshold".

After a marathon, microscopic tears in runners' leg muscles can leak proteins, such as myoglobin, into the bloodstream.

Steel spikes are used to mark the finishing line on athletics tracks and ensure that they are perfectly straight.

Most finishing line tapes are
made from reinforced PVC.

At the 1994 New York Marathon, elite runner Germán Silva took a wrong turn during the final mile and lost his leading position.

However, when he realized his mistake, he returned to the course, chased down his opponent and still won, with a finish time of 2:11:21.